Finally, thanks to Alison Taft and the Creative Writing group organised by the 'Workers Educational Society', Leeds, who gave me the skills and confidence to write this book; and to Ian and Sheila for their support throughout this period.

A percentage of the sales of this book will be donated to Ward 93, St James's Hospital, as well as helping to restore the children's play space in the Bexley wing waiting area.

I0411956

Praise for "Terminal One"

"A moving and uplifting account of the journey involved when coming to terms with a 'terminal' diagnosis. Michael writes from the heart about his experiences from the time of his diagnosis, through a period of denial, then moving on into the treatment prescribed. We also hear the voice of Carole, his wife, as she also struggles to understand and help with their situation. Prepare to laugh and be moved by this heartfelt testimony to life, optimism, and one couple's refusal to quit." *Alison Taft, Tutor and writer, Workers Educational Association, Leeds.*

"A stunning little book - ideal reading for anyone who feels overwhelmed and depressed by their (or their loved one's) medical diagnosis. It's easy to read, written with great humanity and no little skill, and filled with psychological insights and tips for fellow travellers on this most difficult of roads..." *Dr Michael Wilkinson, former Consultant Psychologist and academic tutor for Northern Region Clinical psychology training.*

"A fascinating and moving account of what people go through with a life-shortening illness, written in a unique style and format which is appealing and accessible, helpful and encouraging. It conveys the struggle and denial very well, the uncertainty about the future, frustration, and helplessness; and, lastly, the discomfort of the treatment plan. Balanced by touches of black humour, it approaches the topic in a way which is entertaining, offers hope, and has potential to help others." *Malcolm Henshall, retired teacher.*

ACKNOWLEDGEMENTS

Thanks for the support of Nutricia Advanced Medical Nutrition, who kindly agreed to sponsor the cost of preparing and printing this book; also to Jono Vernon-Powell of Nomadic Thoughts for the superb cover photo, and to Ian Wilkinson and James Nash for help with the editing... without all this help the publication of this book would not have been possible.

Next I would like to express my love and thanks to my partner, Carole for just "being there" through a very difficult period. This story is dedicated to her.

To the wonderful teams of nurses and doctors who have recently won an award for their work with cancer patients in Leeds; I can't thank you enough. Especially: the nurses who work on Ward 93, St James's Hospital, for a splendid job; likewise to the staff on Bexley Wing, and the Radiotherapy Team; the staff of the Robert Ogden Centre based at St James's hospital who offer a warm welcome and counselling in such a comfortable environment; the Macmillan nurses doing a fantastic job in the community; and the staff at Wheatfield's Hospice (in particular 'Andrea', you know who you are!)

Thanks also to the staff at my local pharmacy, 'Mitchell's Chemist' in Horsforth. Last but never least; the recently formed "Rehab Team" who looked after me after my discharge from hospital. Good job, thank you.

I was helped by a mixture of conventional medical treatment for the cancer itself and a range of alternative and complimentary treatments which helped me cope with the symptoms (and the side-effects of the medical treatment). Everyone is different and others will have a different pathway; what helped me may not suit others, and vice-versa. But the important issues are to seek lots of help and advice so that you understand the choices you face, to keep asking questions if you don't understand something, and to face up to the choices you have.

TERMINAL
ONE

Coping with a cancer diagnosis

Michael J Freeman

TERMINAL: being or situated at the end of extremity; (disease) fatal, incurable.
English Dictionary (1996)

First published in Great Britain by Makri press 2015
This edition is an imprint of CreateSpace Independent
Publishing Platform 2015 for sale on Amazon sites and as
a Kindle e-book worldwide

ISBN 978-1-5088277-5-7

Cover image copyright © Jono Vernon-Powell and
Nomadic Thoughts (Worldwide Travel)
Additional design by Makri press

Printed by Createspace

THE AIRPORT

The departure lounge was buzzing and humming with activity; people of all shapes and sizes rushed towards their departure gates, hoping they would not miss their plane. Noises of all kinds came from every direction, interrupted by important announcements about flights to every part of the globe. He nervously glanced at his watch whilst surveying the scene before him. His forehead started to perspire; he asked himself if he had come on the right day. He looked around and wondered if he should ask one of the many faceless people who were passing him by without a second glance. They were all carrying different sizes of baggage, their faces intent and focused on their own destinations and concerns.

"Have I missed the plane?" he asked himself. "Wouldn't be the first time I've arrived at the airport on the wrong day..."

He looked at his watch again. He began to formulate a plan. Usually, he felt he could handle any crisis, but this time it was different. He started to pace around the seating area, feeling like a trapped lion. "I'll not leave my suitcase in case it's confiscated... I'd better pay more attention to the announcements."

He looked at his watch. The clock face appeared to stare at him in disbelief and cry, "Oh no, not again."

He began to search inside his jacket pockets in order to check that his Boarding Pass was still there. For a split second his heart stopped as sweet papers started to litter the floor. He checked his trouser pockets, beginning to panic...

"I'm sure it's here somewhere...?"

* * *

TEDIUM IN THE TERMINAL

He feels alone, standing in the centre of a Terminal,
Sits on a bench; luggage to the right, coffee to the left.
Nothing better to do
But ponder on his thoughts.

His face creases as he listens attentively to the announcements.
Am I staying or leaving?
Many choices to process...
His despair reaches a climax,
So he paces up and down,
Like a tiger in its cage.
He has run out of time
And a decision has to be made.

Other lines of bustling humanity
Start to move towards their destination,
Full of hope combined with trepidation.
They move like giant crocodiles, searching for their prey,
But still his question remains unanswered...
Where do I go now?

*　　*　　*

Out of the background noise, he realises someone is talking to him; as if from a long distance away, he hears the voice of Carole.

"I've written a few poems to expresses my thoughts during this difficult period. Why not include them in the text?"

He thinks for a moment, "That's a great idea, love."

*　　*　　*

"MICHAEL... HEY YOU!"

Bright man;
Bringer of tales to the world;
Tell a tale to me...
Show me an adventure we can try,
Just you and I.
Allow your generous spirit to soar
As we travel our memories.
Your big arms wrapped firmly around my
heart;
Don't let me go yet.

LOOK YOU!
Gregarious man;
A drinker at the feast...
Your preposterous self
Enjoyed a party or two;
Always on the move;
Bar hopping madness;
Seeking out the best ale that you can find...

AND YOU!
Singer of all things musical;
Sing a song to me.
Tell of our mysteries placed in song time;
Create a rhyme of adventure;
Melodic on the ear...

HEY YOU!
Sweet lover of mine;
You found me, amidst the debris of the past.
We found some peace together,
Laughter all the way,
The sun will always shine on you...

*　　*　　*

> ***"If I'd known I was gonna live this long, I'd
> have taken better care of myself."***
> **Eubie Blake, at the age of one hundred**

He was just about to depart for the bar when he thought he heard the flight announcement he was waiting for: "Tomorrow's Airlines regret that flight 564 will be delayed. A further notice will be announced shortly. We apologise for any convenience caused. Any queries will be handled by the Information Desk situated on Level Six."

He checked his ticket, sat back down on his seat and put both his hands around his head. "What should I do? Now it looks as if I'll be late for my appointment. I've been waiting to go for ages. What the hell! I'm going for a pint."

"Don't drink too much. They won't let you on the plane."

His partner's voice echoed through his head as he pushed his way to the front of the bar. "We'll get there eventually," he muttered as he supped his first pint.

"This is Tomorrow's Airlines announcing that flight 565 will be departing in one hour's time. Will all passengers please assemble at Terminal One, Gate 3; Tomorrow's Airline apologise for any inconvenience caused."

His breath was getting unsteady: "I'll just check my Boarding card again." He felt in his inside pockets until he came across the familiar texture of the piece of coloured paper. Nervously he tried to find his Passport. His breathing eased a little as he saw the familiar logo on the cover.

"Better make my way to the gate," he mumbled as he joined the mass of passengers whirling their luggage towards the gates.

*   *   *

Ever felt you are travelling backwards? This is a poem I wrote whilst trying to grasp the reality that I had a problem that I couldn't resolve without help. I felt hopeless and lost, as if I was an explorer in a jungle surrounded by giant weeds that needed clearing...

THE ROAD TO NOWHERE
On the road to nowhere,
Stretching out to a far beyond...
Can't understand why the road is so long.
Don't see any sky in the distance;
So if you insist,
No one will get to the other side.
Somewhere out there
Is where I want to be...
To help reach it,
You must walk faster,
Follow all the guidelines to be safe.
Distance is only a description of measurement;
So if you try harder
You might arrive sooner than you think.
There is no one
To show the way;
You may stray
As you tread the road to nowhere!

*   *   *

He presented his papers to the Air hostess standing at the gate, who smiled at him and everyone else who passed her. He entered the cabin, and after a shuffle he eventually found his seat number: "Just my luck. I've got the middle seat. Hope I'm not sitting next to someone who is always going to the toilet; my worst nightmare."

Just as he got settled, he heard an announcement coming from the aircraft speaker system: "This is your Captain speaking. The airline apologises, but all passengers will have to disembark from the aircraft immediately. There is a technical fault which requires attention. Further announcements will be made soon."

*   *   *

I tried desperately to avoid any treatment. I didn't want to admit I had a problem. But I did visit a local bookshop, and asked Macmillan to send me all their information. The problem was, the more I read, the more determined I became to try and forget about it, because the booklets described all the worst side effects of chemotherapy and radiotherapy...

AVOIDANCE

Know the relationship between man and void.
See the spaces in front...
People who stare and do nothing, become nothing.
Out there you can stop...
Carry on looking out at the void.
Sometimes be a child,
Just waiting for someone to tell you what to do...
Cry, and betray.
Relationships with the void...
It never goes away,
Or moves over, to another place.
Child-like images become frightened and alone,
Seeking a way forward,
Hit out at loved ones.
The brain becomes a fuddled mess
Trying to comprehend how the void works.
Does it ever rest?
Or move to another place?
"Go away!" you plead.
Do not try too hard;
This void may always be stuck in its place,
Waiting for the next move.

*   *   *

He was sitting on the airport bench again. It had been nearly two hours and no announcement had been made. "I'm definitely not going to get to my meeting, now," he thought. "I think I'll make my way to the Information Desk and try and find out what's going on."

He pushed his way towards the desk. Other passengers all crowded around a very small desk. Each person wanted an answer to their query, but most departed looking forlorn and scratching their heads in desperation. One person dressed in a smart uniform was struggling to cope with the sudden rush.

After a long wait he found himself at the front of the queue. "What's happening to flight 565?" he asked nervously.

"We're still awaiting further information, sir," voiced the standard reply.

"Is there any alternative route?" he asked in desperation rather than hope.

"There's a plane departing from another airport, but its fifty miles away. I can get you a seat on it if you wish, compliments of Tomorrow's Airlines."

His brain found it difficult to cope with this new information. "What's the alternative?" he whispered.

"The airline has agreed to give passengers complimentary tickets to the Reality Lounge. Food and drinks are provided there. If you would like to take up that option, I've a couple of tickets left. My guess is that the flight will be postponed and there's likely to be a long wait..."

*　　*　　*

This next poem is how I felt about my husband's illness; I felt that Michael was going to leave me very soon...

GRIEF

Falling, sinking into the abyss of the unknown;
Catch me, I am falling.
Trying to rescue myself,
Seeking out pockets of kindness,
A weeping willow gently bends itself over my lake of tears.
Fluttering shadows of dark and light
Form over the dark water.
Black water brightened by reflections of sun on tree...
Azure sky offers its colour to brighten the mood.
Impenetrable brambles of fear, blocking.

Lift, float, shapes of blossoms,
Those delightful memories
Etching shades of colour
On the canvas of life.

Good day.
Bad day.
Move in different directions each way,
Forming a different mood.
A hand held out to reach,
That which needs gripped tightly,
Scattering emotions.
Ribbons of a river flow every which way,
Undecided as to where to stream;
Diminishing me.

*   *   *

THE REALITY LOUNGE

"Mr Freeman did not wish to discuss prognosis and we therefore have not broached that but we have suggested that he would benefit from getting in touch with the community Macmillan team at this point."

Section of a letter received 4th March, 2013 after the first meeting with the Oral Cancer team.

"Men are disturbed not by what happens to them, but by their opinion of the things that happen..."

Epictetus, a Stoic philosopher (55-135 AD)

The following events took place from November 2013 to April 2014:

In the beginning...

The red lump on the left side of his cheek had grown. "It doesn't feel painful, Carole," he said.

"We better make an appointment with the doctor. It needs checking out," suggested Carole.

"Don't feel that I need to bother anyone. I'm not in any pain."

"We'll go anyway. I'm worried about it."

* * *

They both sat anxiously in the surgery's waiting room, hardly noticing other people who shuffled in and out of the rows of red seats. Their regular doctor wasn't on duty; a locum had replaced her. They were called in to the familiar surroundings of their doctor's room and met by a very friendly, elderly woman who put them at ease with her relaxed approach and manner.

"Have you ever had Mumps as a child?" she asked, as she began the examination.

"I've no idea," he muttered, wondering where this enquiry was going to lead.

"Well my view is that you have caught Mumps and as a consequence you are highly infectious. In your case I have to inform the 'Infectious Disease Department', it's the law now. You'll receive a sample kit in the post in the next couple of days. The kit will make it very clear what you have to do. Meanwhile you best stay in for at least a week."

"Thank you, doctor."

* * *

He rang the surgery: Have the results of my sample arrived yet?"

The receptionist explained that it could take three to four weeks to arrive back, and I would have to wait until Dr Hargreaves arrives back off her holiday, anyway.

"I've been advised to have a check-up at my dentist, Carole. The doctor at the Assessment Unit suggested I should when she sent me home with that course of antibiotics."

"Well it won't harm for them to have a look. We need to try and find out what's happening," said Carole.

* * *

"I don't like the look of that lump, Mr Freeman." (The dentist had just completed her examination.) "I think it might be best if I refer you to the Oral Cancer Clinic and let them examine it as a precaution. I can't find any other problems."

He gulped at the news when he heard those two frightening words; 'oral' and 'cancer'. He couldn't speak for a few minutes.

The dentist's next few words rolled across him like a thick fog: "The clinic will see you very quickly. They don't hang about at the Dental Hospital once they receive a referral."

* * *

"Would you please sit in this chair, Mr Freeman? I need to take a sample from the lump and send it off to the lab." A tall man stood over him waving an instrument around. It had a large needle protruding from the end. He decided to shut his eyes and think of holidays in the Maldives. "This won't take long," he said as he placed the needle inside the lump. He couldn't help but grimace as he felt a sharp pain that lasted for a couple of seconds.

"When will you get the results?" he asked.

"Shouldn't take too long, usually about two weeks, but we'll be in touch."

*   *   *

"I'm afraid the first Biopsy failed to detect anything. I think we'll take a second sample today," said the doctor at their next appointment. Just make yourself comfortable and I'll take another sample."

*   *   *

"It's your heart," explained the specialist in a matter of fact style he found difficult to understand. "It will be a very big risk if we operate but that may be the only way we can get a sample of the tumour…"

He found some difficulty comprehending the real meaning of the situation, and the conversation drifted over him…

"I've had two anaesthetists report that it is too risky to put you to sleep; your heart won't stand the strain of an operation."

He felt his head nodding in full agreement; he wasn't looking forward to going into hospital. He'd been listening to reports from other people about their experiences… and he had a full diary. It would soon be Carole's birthday and the family had booked a week in a farmhouse in Devon. He also had another meeting that evening and couldn't wait to get out of the hospital…

*   *   *

"I'll let the team know that we've failed to get a tissue sample after two tries. I believe you have an appointment in a week's time. I'll refer you for a second MRI scan. Maybe that will tell us if we have missed anything."

*   *   *

He swallowed, and then told Carole: "The results of the MRI scan have shown that there is a massive growth in the neck and lower tongue area. The specialist at the Dental hospital has told me I've got a bad heart, so they won't risk even a small operation to try and get a sample. He would like to get a sample of the tissue, but can't at the moment."

"What shall we do?" asked Carole.

"I wasn't looking forward to being admitted to hospital, so I'm going to forget about it - though I think they want to try another needle biopsy soon." (He has an irrational fear of general anaesthetics based on a dread of not waking up afterwards.)

"You mean we have to sit around that waiting room for another couple of hours?" asked Carole.

"I'm afraid so."

*   *   *

"It looks like a good time to change our life styles. I've also been doing some research into alternative treatments. I'm not happy about receiving radiotherapy."

"Why not?" asked Carole.

"Well, I've been reading about the side effects in the information that Macmillan sent me. I'm going to try and find something else."

*   *   *

I knew I was about to lose my free and easy life; I was very, very reluctant to accept I had a problem. The next poem is a description about how I felt at the time; I was hopeful that I could find an alternative treatment that would not include radiotherapy or chemotherapy.

EXPERIENCES OF FREEDOM

Does freedom die?
Or continue to live within a flame of uncertainty?
Begging the question,
A flame leaps out and burns...
This hurts!

So stand back, think of better times.
The pain disappears,
Feelings start to drag.

A runaway train approaches, rattling down the track...
Trapped on the rail;
Begin to panic, shouting for help, crying out for freedom.
With others to aid,
The train slows down,
Our flame stops.

Togetherness brings its own closeness,
Helping drive the demons away!
Make way for a future
That has ingredients,
Hope, love, and the power of the divine...?

*　*　*

"You know it's easy to blame myself for this," he remarked.

"Why, for God's sake?" shouted Carole.

"I joined the Navy at fifteen and a half, too much beer and rum, if you ask me."

"Don't be daft. I read about a footballer, who has the same symptoms as you. This could happen to anyone."

*   *   *

"We've got a weekend in Glastonbury coming next week. I've managed to book you a session with Daisy on the Saturday afternoon. You got some benefit last time you went." Carole was busily flicking through her diary.

"That 'Vortex Healing' seems to be very powerful. The last session helped me to relax and Daisy said that I could heal myself."

He was looking forward to escaping for the weekend. He was holding a letter from the oncologist which gave him the date for his next appointment. This was getting serious...

In the UK, Glastonbury is a major centre for alternative and complementary medicines. Many are based on Eastern beliefs about energy and spirituality that support the body's innate or natural healing abilities. Health experts agree that there is no evidence for their effectiveness, but neither are they likely to be harmful as long as they are not used to replace conventional care or to postpone seeing a health care provider. In the USA, studies have shown that religious and spiritual values are important in how patients and caregivers cope with the anxiety caused by diseases like cancer.

*   *   *

"I've been reading a book on cancer that we bought from Waterstones, it's by Rosy Daniels. She is a very easy read," he said.

"Go on. Has it been useful?" asked Carole.

"It suggests a charity that will offer information on alternative treatments. I think they'll provide me with funding to pay for a telephone conversation with a qualified nurse. Her name is Patricia Peat." He was excited about this discovery.

The UK website www.yestolife.org.uk offers free support and lifestyle advice for cancer sufferers and arranges consultations on alternative and complementary treatments for a small charge (grants available, dependent on circumstances).
In the US, the National Center for Complementary and Integrative Health (NCCIH) is the Federal Government's lead agency for scientific research on complementary and integrative health approaches. Their website www.nccih.nih.gov is a great source of information about complementary health products and practices.

"Patricia has told me about a Consultant based at London University College Hospital. He is offering a treatment that sounds similar to Laser Beams," he said.

"What's his name?" asked Carole.

"Mr Colin Hooper, apparently he's the world leader in photodynamic therapy for head and neck cancer. It's mainly used with people who can't have radiotherapy - not really a cure but it can slow things up. But it does offer fewer side effects as you are only in hospital for five days. I would obviously have to travel to London, but I'm not sure how practical that will be?"

Colin Hooper: Consultant at University College Hospital, London. Photodynamic therapy, an alternative treatment for some head and neck cancers, is not currently funded by the NHS. In the US, the National Cancer Institute is the primary source for all information about

cancer detection, diagnosis, treatment, prevention, control and palliative care (www.cancer.gov). They have a factsheet about photodynamic therapy, and also provide a general information service by phone, webchat or email at: www.cancer.gov/aboutnci/cis

"We could ask your oncologist what he feels about it when we see him next week," suggested Carole. "But maybe it's worth a try."

*　　*　　*

When you hear the word: "cancer" your mind drifts about all over the place. I didn't know which way to turn, so I wrote this poem:

THE PENDULUM

Round and heavy,
Moving left, and then right,
Never ceasing, nor ending...
Which way will it fall?
Watch it carefully.
Moving swiftly,
Ticking time away...
Will it end, or descend,
on a pathway that is clear?
Blow life away?
When the mind is such a mystery,
Can it help, to yelp?
A cry... (for help!)

The brass levers always move;
Gravity takes over,
So we need a four leaf clover,
Pointing towards our destiny.
Take it, leave it?
Descend and catch a cloud, fly away.

Leave this pendulum alone
To make its own tone...
Stop in the middle,
Try and solve the riddle...
Please tell me it will rest,
Do your best...
This pendulum's still there.

* * *

"You're surely not thinking about not having any treatment?" his daughter cried.

"It did cross my mind a couple of times," he replied softly.

"What's the alternative if you don't do something? My guess is that the tumour will spread and you'll die."

"I had thought of that. But I've been reading about the side effects and they are horrendous."

"You'll be fine. You're fit and well, so there shouldn't be much problem. Besides my baby will be here soon and my guess is that you will want to be part of her life."

"I'll give it some serious thought, love. Carole has said the same."

Palliative: alleviating without curing
"English Dictionary (2000)

The reality of the contents of the letter had slowly sunk in. Although it appeared to be a terminal diagnosis he was a practical man and, therefore, decided to make the appropriate arrangements. He asked: "Do you think it's a good idea to alter our bank accounts, so the finances are in your name?"

Carole nodded. "But our savings may not be enough, so if you go I'll struggle to pay for a funeral," screamed an anxious Carole.

"We better start stashing some spare cash away," he suggested.

* * *

It cost a lot of money to pay a Solicitor to arrange 'Power of Attorney'.

"We've got to prepare for the worst. I don't want to leave you in a mess", he said. "If I'm seriously ill you can sign all the relevant forms and get money from the accounts. Les, our finance advisor, has also promised to review our mortgage, under the circumstances. So we can access more cash if needed."

"But we haven't to go mad," suggested Carole. "I don't want piles of debt if anything happens to you."

"But I've always wanted to go to Las Vegas,"

"It will be too hot and expensive, but we'll look into it next time we are in town."

* * *

"I think I'd better contact Robert Ogden Centre and see if they have a counsellor free, Carole," he was worried. "They helped me a lot last time I had Cancer."

"That's not a bad idea. It will help you make sense of what's going on," replied Carole.

The Robert Ogden Macmillan Cancer Information and Support Centre at St James Hospital, Leeds, offers a comfortable and friendly space for anyone living with cancer and their relatives and friends. The centre offers information, social and counselling services, practical help and complementary therapies, and group classes and programmes to help people manage their own health problems. It is a great example of integrative medicine, in which care is tailored to the individual and focuses on health maintenance, prevention, education, environment, and the body's innate ability to heal itself, in conjunction with conventional treatment.

* * *

He picked up the phone which had sent a piercing ring through his lounge. "Hello," said a soft female voice. "My name is Andrea and I'm a Palliative Nurse and I've been asked to contact you. When will it be convenient to visit?"

The word 'palliative' didn't register.

"I am based at Wheatfield's Hospital, perhaps you have heard of it?" The voice sounded reassuring and he began to relax.

There were many questions flashing in his mind, but he couldn't speak as the reality of the introduction became to sink in. He did mumble a time and day after checking his diary.

"I'm not dying, am I, Carole?"

"Not as far as I know, but the doctors did explain that we would need to make the necessary preparations. When is the nurse coming?"

"Next Tuesday at 10.30, are you free?" he asked.

Palliative care is care given to improve the quality of life of patients who have a serious or life-threatening disease. The aims are to prevent or treat as early as possible the symptoms of a disease, the side effects caused by treatment, and the psychological, social, and spiritual problems related to the disease.

She walked into his lounge and her presence and demeanour soon made him feel relaxed. Andrea began carefully to describe her role, "I explained on the phone that the Hospice has had a referral from the hospital. So it's my job to provide you with all the support I can."

"Can you explain your role?" he asked.

"Of course; I've read all your notes sent to me by the specialist at the Dental Hospital, so this is an initial assessment visit when we'll work out a plan that will, hopefully, support you and Carole."

He said, "I like the idea of going into a Hospice, especially if I'm very ill. I don't like being fully dependant on Carole looking after me at home. I want to feel comfortable, but not go into hospital."

Carole asked, "Is there a bed available at the Hospice?"

"Yes, there will be no problem", she answered.

"Is it possible to visit?" he asked tentatively, his tone of voice betraying the fact that the reality of his situation had not sunk in.

"It's too early to think about that. You can be sure these things can easily be arranged later." Her smile defused the strained atmosphere.

"I've been doing some research into other treatments as I don't like the idea of taking the traditional route," he explained. It was on his mind, so he had to talk about it. "You see I've got a serious heart problem, so I can't have any operations. I feel happy about this. I wasn't looking forward to an operation."

Andrea said: "There'll be someone from the office who deals with benefits."

"Pardon?" he said, surprised. "What benefits are those?"

"Ross will explain it all when she rings; your diagnosis entitles you to claim Attendance Allowance."

Attendance Allowance is a welfare benefit given in the UK to help with the costs of personal care for people with serious and disabling conditions (amount depends on circumstances.)

The phone call came the next day. Ross explained that she'd take care of everything. He would receive 'special treatment' which would fast forward his application and he would receive a Blue Parking Badge.

Macmillan Cancer Support is a major UK charity (www.macmillan.org.uk) which funds nurses and other staff and builds cancer care centres in conjunction with the National Health Service. They also provide information and offer toll-free telephone support (Mon to Fri 9am to 8pm) on 0808 808 0000 The equivalent in the USA is the American cancer society (www.cancer.org) who offer 24

Andrea returned two weeks later.

He began to explain: "Well, as they can't get a sample from the mass that is there, I thought I'd try an alternative plan. I've received some information by contacting an organisation called 'Cancer Options' and I managed to receive some funding from 'Yes to Life'. This organisation offers advice on alternative treatments." He was quite excited about discovering information that would lead him away from the radiotherapy couch. His denial was complete!

"Go on," Andrea sounded empathic, which gave him the confidence he needed.

He explained, "I've recently been on the phone to an advisor who is part of 'Cancer Options'. She has done lots of research. Her name is Patricia Peat and she has offered me an alternative route which might be appropriate and it produces fewer side effects."

"I've not come across anything that's better than radiotherapy," Andrea explained.

"Well, I've found out about this consultant who works at the London University College Hospital and he's pioneered a treatment called 'Photo dynamic therapy'. It could be compared to Laser treatment. My oncologist doesn't think I'll be eligible for the treatment, but I thought it would be worth a try."

"What's his name?" asked Andrea.

"Mr Colin Hooper, he's on holiday at the moment, so I can't get any information."

"Must be frustrating, I guess? But if you're offered another biopsy, it might be worth considering. At least you'll know what we're dealing with"

He said reluctantly, "I'll consider it, Andrea. Thanks for the suggestion."

*   *   *

I was going through a very anxious time, especially when I was informed that the doctor couldn't get a sample of the tissue. The long needle biopsy also failed to provide a sample.

THE ANXIOUS CLOUD

The anxious cloud,
Shouting out loud...

I came across this cloud quite suddenly.
I first saw it as it blocked the sun.
To dismiss… not me, surely...

This cloud was unappealing,
Never disappearing,
Frightening in its own unique way.
Sometimes I needed to scream;
I thought it was a nightmare; would never end.

I became lost in this particular thought,
Seeking a way forward,
Not knowing how this cloud would react,

I asked a question.
The cloud failed to answer.
Every day I saw the cloud;
I could only stare at its grinning face
Never moving from the same place.

*   *   *

Andrea returned three weeks later; Carole had asked to meet her alone.

Carole cried, "How long has he got?"

"I simply can't answer that question,"

"Will he choke to death?"

"No, that won't happen."

"When will he be admitted to the Hospice?"

"It's early days yet."

"I don't know what to do."

"Just carry on as you are. You seem to be doing a splendid job. I can see that you are upset."

"Yes, I am. I feel so helpless."

"It is hard for the carers, probably harder than for the patients."

"I'm beginning to realise that. He seems oblivious to what's happening."

"It's not unusual for this to happen. Don't forget I'm only a phone call away."

* * *

"Are you coming with me to see my heart doctor, Carole?" he asked.

"Yes, of course, we're in this together. I expect we'll be waiting hours, again," replied Carole.

"Well it's best to see what he has to say. He has known me a lot longer than the two people who claim my heart won't stand an operation."

"We'll never find anywhere to park. All the disabled bays will be full," said Carole.

"But we need to explore other treatment options. That's if there are any," he remarked.

* * *

He was greeted like an old friend: "Sit down Mr Freeman. It's nice to see you and your good lady. How are you both?" asked Dr Smith.

He became instantly relaxed as he settled into one of the chairs in front of a large wooden desk. He had been coming to see Dr Smith for many years and knew him to have a five star rapport with all his patients.

"Apparently my heart won't survive an operation. They need to get a tissue sample, so they can decide on a treatment plan," he explained.

"Let me think," Dr Smith rubbed his cheek whilst moving over to the screen on his office computer. "I can see clearly what has happened," he remarked. "I think the best way forward is to refer you for a couple of tests. Let's see if we can convince them to rethink."

"What kind of tests?" he asked nervously.

"One involves riding a bike whilst attached to an oxygen mask. It doesn't take too long. The other involves you collecting a small machine from downstairs that will measure your breathing at night time. When all the results come though, we'll meet again to work out our next move. It's nice to see you both again. Don't worry we'll try and get something sorted out." Dr Smith held out his long arm to signal that the consultation was over.

He left feeling much better.

*   *   *

"Explain what Reiki is, Carole. I've always wanted to know."

Carole replied: "Reiki is a Japanese term for 'Universal Life Energy'. It refers to the unseen energy that underlies all life and flows through everything that lives. As a healer I'm attuned to this energy so I can channel it to others who attend a healing session. It is important that my Clients are relaxed and willing to accept the process; otherwise the energy can be blocked. There are many systems; the one I practise is just called 'Usui Reiki'. I place my hands on what are called the 'Chakra Centres' which are basic energy centres in the body; everyone has them. The treatment can take up to one hour, but my sessions are usually forty five minutes. During this time I take my energy which has arrived from the Universe and pass it to my client. I have some evidence that the treatments work as clients return to me for more sessions. I believe that the process links the body on all levels; physical, emotional and spiritual. There are seven chakras, with openings into the energy points within the physical body. Each Chakra vibrates at a different energy when opened and balanced. When any of the chakras are closed or blocked, disease can occur. One of the things I'll be doing when I heal you is to correct the problem and try and clear any clogged or blocked chakras which will allow Reiki energy to flow freely into your body."

"When I went to see Daisy in Glastonbury what was happening to me?"

"You mean what is 'Vortex Healing'?"

"Yes," he replied.

"Vortex Healing is similar, but a relatively new energy healing process which uses the 'KI' or 'CHI' system, a more dramatic form of energy processed through a Healer who has been attuned and highly experienced. The Healer will often use sounds of their voice to tune into the client. The Clients will probably require several sessions before they feel any benefits."

"That sounds very mystical and mysterious."

"Maybe, but for me it's normal, like religion is for other people. I believe that being a healer is a 'Way of Being' or a calling. It's just how I am, everywhere I go."

*　　*　　*

I spent a lot of time daydreaming. I was in denial and wanted to get away as far as possible. Let me catch a bus; any bus would do.

THE BUS TOUR

You feel you are on a no 39 bus going down a steep hill.
This bus has no brakes or gears.
Such are my fears.

A picture formed in the window,
Displays a wealth of beautiful countryside;
This now helps to guide my thoughts
Towards a more comfortable place.

Just after a meal,
When stomach aches and churns,
You hope the bus will come to a stop at the bottom of a hill.
Let's hope!
Let's hope!

*   *   *

"Let's book a holiday," he suggested.

"I've been looking at Croatia. Looks very nice," said Carole.

"I feel great at the moment, so I won't bother with shopping around for travel insurance. We'll just have to risk it. It's only for two weeks."

* * *

"I think we'd better book you in for a second scan," the doctor looked at him with a stern expression. "We can then compare it with your first scan. Be good to see if there is anything that has changed."

He explained, "Whilst on holiday I began to develop a cough and a nasty sore throat, so I thought it best to try and do something."

"Not before time. We really don't want to leave it too long," sighed the doctor.

He was slowly moving into the real world. The illness on holiday had given him the signal. Carole convinced him he would have to act.

* * *

The couple had waited two hours for an appointment. They were both tired and worried. They had entered the state of the art building which had sprung up only five years ago. The waiting areas were very comfortable, lots of comfy chairs scattered around. He noticed a TV had been placed in one corner and a pile of second hand books took over another. There were plenty of tables scattered around the room. It had a warm, cosy feeling about it as hospital staff buzzed around completing their various tasks.

The hospital waiting room was now getting depressingly familiar, but a routine was settling in. A coffee morning was being advertised and he noticed that the date would be after his last appointment. They decided to have two goes on the 'Guess the name of the teddy' as it somehow gave them a small boost. It was a flashback to normality.

"I've listed a few questions for the oncologist, Carole." He had found a section in Rosy Daniel's book and received some ideas from a couple of friends.

"Let me see," said Carole.

What is the exact name of the cancer?
How long has the cancer been there?
How big is it?
Is it localized?
Has the cancer left its primary site?
Is it likely to be a primary or a secondary type?
What stage is it?
How fast it is growing now?
How aggressive is the tumour?
Will the tumour grow more slowly or faster at different stages?
Do these tumours sometimes stop growing spontaneously and what are the dangers if it doesn't?
What are the recommended treatments and how do they work?
How long will this take and who would give it?
What will happen if I do nothing?
Would it be detrimental to postpone?
Once the treatment is finished what are the chances of it coming back?
Could I get a second opinion, if so how?

EXIT AHEAD

"The mass hasn't got any bigger. You can have a glance on this screen if you wish," suggested the doctor. "If you look carefully, you can clearly see that there is a small malignancy growing near your left Lymph Gland. It demonstrates that the cancer is spreading." The doctor looked at him, gesturing him to get closer to the screen. Prior to this he had been afraid to look at this imposing object floating around his upper body, like a giant Jelly Fish.

"I can see it. You must be able to see it?" Carole said, frustrated at the turn of events. She began to wipe away a tear.

"Because the Tumour seems nearer will there be a better chance of getting a sample?" he asked, feeling a little shocked at this new development.

"I was just about to make that suggestion. I'll book you in for a second needle biopsy. You shouldn't have to wait long."

*   *   *

"Shall we get together and have a meditation?" asked Carole.

He replied, "Think that might be good as I'm having that second biopsy. I'll choose one of your crystals as well."

"I think that's a brilliant idea."

"I'll take one of the crystals with me when I go for the biopsy."

*   *   *

The oncologist looked at the couple in front of him after examining the screen perched on his desk: "It confirms that it is a malignant tumour and one that's going to cause you problems if we don't do something about it. It's definitely cancer and a high grade, so now we know."

He looked stunned and could hardly speak. His mouth had gone dry. Carole began to cry softly, trying desperately to suppress her tears.

Somehow he managed to squeeze out some words: "What happens next?"

"I'll arrange an appointment for you to come in and have a mask made as I'm going to recommend that you have thirty-four doses of radiotherapy. I don't think it will be wise to offer chemotherapy as well, based on your current heart condition."

He found his enquiring mind suddenly kicking into a fourth gear, "Why do I have to have thirty four sessions?"

"Good question," the oncologist smiled reassuringly. It's been proved over time that this amount of treatment will work. You'll have to take my word for it."

He uttered a sigh of relief. He hadn't been looking forward to receiving both radiotherapy and chemotherapy. He found it difficult to understand how anyone could survive the ongoing side effects of having both treatments at the same time.

Carole had composed herself and asked, "How soon will the treatment start?"

"Within the next two weeks," came the swift reply." The nurse will look after you and give you all the details. Don't worry. We're here to keep an eye on you all through the treatment plan. I'll see you in the first week once the radiotherapy starts. The doctor stood up and held out his hand. "I feel there is a good chance of a cure, now we know where to target. So don't worry."

*   *   *

I was worried about receiving treatment. These are my thoughts at the time. I'm a person who likes to try and be practical. But it doesn't always work out like that, does it?

RAGING HEART

The heart is now in a complete rage.
It reflects a strange mixture of responses;
The inner stomach aches to pray for forgiveness,
Let's feel for those who are in pain.

Like the prisoner searching for the key to a cell.
You wish you could ring the bell
And together fire an arrow of joy
From lost soul to desolate planet...

To Highway 66...
To fast forward...
To the strength of the individual,
Trying to square the circle.

The heart then repeats a sound
That can live "to be" for another day.

*　　*　　*

MASQUARADE

"What's happening today?" asked Carole.

He replied, "I'm having a mask made apparently. You don't need to come to this if you need a break."

"I'm coming, so I know what's going on."

"Thanks, love. I could do with the company."

"What's this mask look like?" asked Carole.

"Well they cover all your face with this plaster, although it's not like real plaster. It seems to have a different texture. They are very precise and it fits tightly on all your face. They asked me if I would like eye slits cut out. I said yes, if it was more comfortable."

*   *   *

"What's it all for?"

"It helps the radiologist target the right area. When the mask dried, they did a dummy run. It felt very uncomfortable, but I've been told I'll get used to it, eventually. The mask will ensure that the beams will target the same place. It will hold my head down to a large bench situated under the radiation machine which is lined up by making a series of tattoo marks scratched onto parts of my body. I suppose there are worse things than lying on a flat board trapped by a tight fitting mask listening to three complete strangers shouting out numbers. But I guess they know what they're doing."

"I hope so."

*   *   *

The list looked daunting. His counsellor at the Robert Ogden Centre suggested he cross off all the dates as he went along. This list represented an account of all the dates for the thirty four visits to the radiotherapy department. It seemed very imposing and was to rule their life for the duration.

"Look at this, Carole our whole life is now planned for us."

"Let me see it, please? Hmmm...they've included visits to see the oncologist every week, just as he promised. You've also appointments with a nurse and a dietician. We'll certainly be well looked after."

"Let's hope so," he sighed. "I think we are going to need it."

*   *   *

"Isn't it a nice place?"

"There are lots of nice comfortable chairs to sit in," Carole remarked.

"I have to go to the next waiting room. I'm assigned to 'Linac 10' machine. Follow me, love."

"Just take a seat anywhere you can," ordered the secretary sat behind a large desk. "If there any delays they'll be announced on the screen over on the wall, so it's best to keep an eye out."

He looked despondently at the screen, hardly noticing the adverts that flashed on and off. He sighed when he saw the notice: "Linac 10 delayed one hour."

"We're in for a long wait. Better get out your crossword, love."

*   *   *

I felt so sorry for Michael when he had his mask fitted. I tried to imagine what it was like for him wearing it every day for weeks and endless weeks.

THE MASK

Hold on tight
Bring me down softly
From this disordered violence of disease
Place me in that moulded mask
Bolt me down
Kill the cells
Don't kill me

Hold still
Don't move
Allow the sickening rays to heal
Don't let the fear overtake me
Tumbling nightmares envelope me
The dark tunnel awaits;
I am spiralling down

Keep me safe
During this turmoil
Mixing the emotions
From believing in the inevitable
To finding a miracle
Intertwining anguish with hope

*   *   *

"What was it like?" Carole asked.

He replied, "Well they show you into this small waiting room where you have to put on one of those gowns. They hardly fit. Then you wait for a short while before someone knocks on the door and escorts you down a long corridor. The first thing you see is a large picture of purple Lilacs growing in a field. I thought they might help me relax a little, I was so nervous."

"Then what happens?"

"I had to lie down on a bench. My mask was waiting for me at the top. I decided to call it Fred."

"Fred? What kind of name is that?"

"Well it looks like a Fred."

* * *

Tony had been part of their family for a long time; fostered as a child, now an adult they cared for. Until his treatment had actually started, Tony hadn't really understood that Michael was ill. But he did now.

"Only thirty-three more to go," moaned Carole.

"They are running two hours late today, love. Do you think you will be able to get back home in time for Tony returning from the Centre?"

"We'll see how it goes. Sometimes they can be quicker than that board says."

"I guess we'll just have to get used to it. One of the machines has broken down."

"They're always breaking down. We've been very unlucky this last week. Yesterday we sat here for three hours. I'm fed up."

"Well at least I'm being treated, which wasn't going to happen a few weeks ago."

"Yes, there's always a positive side. Let's hope it's worth it."

"Tony has been upset at his Day Centre. They have just rung," explained Carole. "I think he's very worried about you."

"I'll have another word with him when he gets home. I expect he's feeling mixed up about what's going on," he replied.

* * *

"Are you OK, Tony?" he asked. "I've nearly finished my treatment and I'm not so bad at the moment." He watched Tony thinking hard. It really was like watching a child in a man's body.

"What's happening tomorrow?" asked Tony.

"I've got to have more treatments. They put me under a big machine, but it's only for a short while. It doesn't hurt."

"I'll look after you if you want," suggested Tony.

"No, I'll be alright; try and settle at the Day Centre. I'll let you know how I get on."

"Thanks, Michael. I'll go get my tablets now before I have a shower."

"Tony is very worried about you," said Carole, watching him climb the stairs.

* * *

"When are you going to Disney Land, Keith?" he asked. He had decided to get to know as many names of the staff as possible. It became a 'survival' tactic. Yesterday he had had a long conversation with one of the female radiologists who had informed him she was getting married. He suggested she contact his stepson's hotel. The hotel arranged weddings at very reasonable rates. Deborah smiled at his suggestion and explained that she was going to check on a few venues over the weekend. He asked her to let him know how she got on.

"To answer your question," Keith replied, "I'm going tomorrow for a couple of weeks. Can you move your right shoulder a little to the left? Inch down the bed a little whilst I fit the mask. It looks like you've lost weight, so I'll have to readjust the clamps."

He felt as if he was an extra in the film 'Iron Man' as the mask was clamped down tight over his face. He was grateful for the friendly banter between himself and the staff, some of whom he had made an effort to get to know better. He felt like a stranger when he was sent to another machine.

Once the staff left, he would try and relax and listen to the music on one of the CDs he had brought in. That's if the staff remembered to switch the sound up. He had started to feel uncomfortable when the mask was finally fitted, as he could hardly breathe due to spittle forming in the back of his throat. He tried desperately not to think about this by concentrating on the music, which had to compete with all the strange sounds that came out of the machine and whirled around just above his head.

It often reminded him of scenes from 'Dr Who' or 'Star Trek'.

* * *

"I feel terrible, Carole."

"Why, what's up?"

"The Dietician wants me to put on some weight and I'm having problems getting all the supplement drinks down me. I've also got to take loads of medications. There's never time in the day."

"We'll see what the oncologist says tomorrow."

* * *

He practically crawled into the consulting room.

The oncologist appeared to read his mind; one of the nurses looked sympathetically at him as he flopped down on a chair. A quiet, but stern voice began to explain that the last ten treatments should now take place in hospital; this was now the best option. "I predicted this would happen," the doctor commented, as he handed a piece of paper to the nurse.

* * *

WARD 93

He wasn't in any position to argue. His resistance to being admitted to hospital had disappeared like so much straw in the wind. Score: treatment six, body nil. In tennis terms it was game, set and match. Within a few hours he was escorted by Carole to Ward 93. This small four bed compound was to be his home for the next ten days.

"This is a very friendly ward," a Welsh sounding voice boomed from the bed opposite. "All the staff will look after you."

"Let's settle you in," suggested Carole who started to unpack some of his belongings. "I'll buy you some new pyjamas. It looks like you're going to need them."

"We need to take your blood pressure," a young lad not much older than his son stood before him pushing a small machine. "You'll have to have this done every four hours."

* * *

"I've got to put a saline drip in," ordered a stern looking nurse who soon began to dig a needle into his left wrist. "You need fluids by the looks of it."

He had decided to submit to anything. His body had admitted total defeat. "I'll just lie here and think of nice things. Perhaps see what's on the TV, after I put some credits in."

* * *

"Hello, my name is Sue. There are two Sues on this ward. How are you feeling?" He looked up from his bed and felt a sigh of relief as he was greeted by a friendly looking nurse who began to assemble a variety of instruments spread out on a small trolley. "I'm going to fit a feeding tube. We need to get some calories down you. It won't take long. The good news is that we can put all your different medications through the tube. Makes life a lot easier and it won't hurt a bit."

Sue had a manner about her that he could instantly trust. "I'm on duty for the next twelve hours, so if you need anything just press the buzzer that's just behind you. Just try and sit up for a few minutes whilst I fit this tube."

*   *   *

"You've got a tube up your left nostril," remarked Carole.

"It's not as bad as it looks. You get used to it after a while. The nurse was very good at fitting it and once it's in there aren't many problems. It's a lot easier getting all the medication down me."

"Your brother wants to visit over the weekend. Jackie and Derek will also be coming," said Carole.

"That's nice of them. They could help transport all this gear I've been given. Otherwise it could take us ages," he said as he glanced around at the stack of boxes that contained his feeding tube and stand.

*   *   *

"What's the time?" he asked as he pushed the large metal stand towards the toilet. He was trying desperately not to trip over the feeding tube that was hanging precariously from a point on the stand. He knew it would not be a pleasant task replacing the tube that he had become totally reliant on. His sleep had been disturbed by a need to go to the toilet as well as his throat beginning to ache.

He had also begun to master the art of keeping ahead of the pain; he was always relieved when the nurse arrived with the painkiller. "Hello?"

"It's three in the morning," came the soft reply from behind the desk which dominated the nurse's station, hardly visible in the dim light.

"Please can I have some more morphine? My throat is killing me."

"I'll be over in a minute."

*   *   *

40

"Hello, my name is Jane. I'm part of a team of dieticians looking after you. I'll help decide how much food you're going to need through the tube once you are discharged. You'll be going home in a couple of days. The staff will make sure you can feed yourself and teach you how to administer all your meds. I hear you are doing well with that. But keep practising won't you?"

"Thank you, I think I'm getting the hang of it," he croaked. He was finding it difficult to speak.

"I've seventeen different medicines to take over the course of the day, Carole."

He was perched in his arm chair which had become a familiar place for him to spend the majority of his time. "And I'm being sent home with three boxes of food plus all the gear that goes with it. Can you arrange for some help?"

"Jackie will help us," replied Carole. "You'll be coming home soon."

"Can't wait, I've been looked after very well, but I am getting fed up of being woken up in the middle of the night just so they can take my blood pressure. Must be a good reason for this otherwise they wouldn't do it."

"We're all going to stay at Daniel's hotel over Christmas. Do you think you'll be fit enough to go?" asked Carole.

"That will be something to look forward to," he nodded. "I won't be eating any Christmas dinner, though."

*   *   *

This is my way of thanking all the staff who work on Ward 93. I was dreading going into hospital, but the experience made me realise just how hard the medical and nursing professions work. It was definitely a case of what doesn't kill you makes you stronger.

TRIBUTE TO WARD 93

Spare a thought my friends,
For those who care;
Who work long hours
And never lose their smiles
Like flowers in full bloom.

To witness dedication is a privilege;
Whilst completing arduous tasks
Full of contentment and charm,
A pleasing scene for those in strife.

Pounding feet interrupt my thoughts,
Serious faces stare down,
Brush away the pain
With their reassuring voices,
Before tending to others
Not far away.

So farewell to those who put other people first.
I will never forget their kindness,
All the care that came in waves.

So I rest my pen,
In the hope
This tribute will suffice.

*　*　*

"Look at all the meds. We're going to have to be organised. Not sure where I'm going to put them all." He had left the safe confines of Ward 93 and was now in his study at home surrounded by cardboard boxes full of liquid food and lots of bottles and packets of medication. "Have to check all the times on each bottle. There are four types of painkillers to start with."

"I feel like we are in a chemist," remarked Carole. "Let's put them all on your old computer desk. Then we can see what's what. And what does that sheet tell us?"

"It's a full list of all the meds. It includes the dosage and frequency of each one. We will have to take our time reading all the directions before we can get our heads around it." He placed the three pages on top of the desk. "They told me to ring up the ward if there are any problems. I don't know if I'll get much joy on a Friday night."

"A nurse from that company they told us about on the ward is coming to see me tomorrow, Carole."

"What's she coming for?"

"To train me up on the art of using this tube; I must ask her how this rucksack works," he replied as he started to unpack some of the equipment and food that had just been delivered.

"I'll keep everything in the spare bedroom. I'd hate to think what people do who only have a small flat. The boxes of food take up a lot of space and I've two boxes of spare tubes and syringes."

"I'm not sure I'm using the pump correctly. I have to be careful when I go to the toilet during the night. I'm terrified that I'll pull my tube out. Don't fancy having to have another fitted."

The Nurse from 'Fresenius Kabi' arrived promptly the next morning. She explained that the rucksack could easily take the place of the metal stand, especially at night time. He scratched his head in bewilderment as he witnessed the Nurse weaving the tube through the cut out channels fitted in the rucksack. He made a cheeky mental note never to use this method unless he had to, although it would be easier to use if he had to stay somewhere overnight. She also demonstrated that he had been using the metal stand incorrectly.

"Easy when you know how," he remarked. "That will make my life easier."

'Fresenius Kabi' is a global health care company that specialises in lifesaving medicines and technologies for infusion, transfusion and clinical nutrition. It is used by the NHS in the UK to provide Home Care to people who have been discharged from hospital and require tube feeding; they have a nationwide team of Nurse Advisors who work alongside hospitals and dieticians to provide 24hour care and advice. The company provides the liquid food and equipment needed for tube feeding, and 24hr telephone support from a trained Nurse.

* * *

"I've just had a coughing fit, Carole. That tube is hanging out of my mouth. What shall we do? Shall we ring for an ambulance?" He was shaking and sweating as he had run down the stairs in order to get some help. In the middle of putting all his medication down the tube he had started to cough. The tube suddenly finished up hanging just outside his lips. It was a strange sensation and he panicked.

"Let's ring Ward 93 first," suggested Carole.

"Good thinking," he replied finding himself calming down a little.

"The nurse I spoke to suggests you go to Bexley Wing straight away. I'll drive you," suggested Carole.

The Nurse on duty on the Ward soon helped by explaining that all they had to do is cut the tube with a pair of scissors. "You can then just pull the rest and it will come out of your nose very easily.   I'll have to fit a new tube. They are very thin and fragile, so be prepared to have a few fitted if necessary. Let's hope in your case it won't be. Just remind me of your date of birth."

"I don't like it when the tube is fitted," he turned around on the bed in the waiting room to face the Nurse who was getting prepared to fit the new tube. He took a deep breath.

"This won't take long. Which nostril do you prefer?"

"The last one went relatively easily up my left one," he replied as he started to swallow. His eyes started to water and he gripped his hands in his fingers as the nurse expertly fitted the tube back through his nostril and down to his stomach.

"I'll have to test it to see if it's in the right place. You may have to go to X ray if there's a problem." He groaned at the thought of having to get to the X ray department which was situated on the other side of the hospital. The nurse fitted a syringe on a point in the tube. The main reason for this he had been informed was to make sure the tube had rested in the right place inside his stomach. He had had to complete this same test every time he had a feed or took his medication. He knew that if the sample taken from his stomach did not produce the correct colour then there had to be a delay. If this occurred at home he would have to abandon the feed whilst he lay down on his bed making sure he was positioned on his right side.

A helpful nurse on Ward 93 also suggested he clean his teeth and/or gargle. He was also advised to take some exercise by walking up and down the stairs. Thankfully, he found that both of these options worked and he could gain the correct result when he placed a sample of liquid from his stomach onto the test patches. He found this procedure quite frustrating at times, but it had to be done as there was a danger that he could flood his lungs which would simulate drowning. Not a pleasant thought!

*   *   *

"Merry Christmas," he said as he greeted his extended family who had arrived at the hotel managed by his stepson Daniel. He'd taken the decision to attend the annual festivities over a week ago and in spite of what had occurred beforehand he didn't feel too bad.

Everyone sat in a circle in the Hotel bar as they exchanged presents. He smiled as he watched the joy on the faces of two of the younger children who seemed intent on building a den with the chairs and tables. Soon it was time to go into the large and comfortable dining room to have a traditional Christmas dinner. He decided to sit down at the end of the elaborately decorated table and witness the arrival of some of the seven course meal.

After a few courses had been served he suddenly remembered that he had forgotten to bring a vital piece of equipment. He felt he had no choice but to return home. This would be no problem as he had had no alcohol to drink.

"I won't be too long, Carole. I've forgotten my feeding tube."

The party was in full swing when he re-joined the family who were in the middle of a quiz game. "What are you playing?" he asked "Can you move that table so I can put this metal feeding stand on it. It will give it some height. I know the answer to that question."

"Don't shout it out, it's a team game and we're losing," Carole said.

"Happy New year," someone shouted.

*   *   *

"That bloody tube has come out again, Carole. I'll have to ring Ward 95 as it's the weekend." He had had another coughing fit which resulted in the tube protruding through his mouth. This time he didn't panic and quickly used a pair of scissors which he always kept handy near his medication as they were very useful for opening packets of medicine.

"Ok, but I'm busy here. Can you manage to get yourself there? If you need any help then I'll come and pick you up."

"I'll be fine. I don't feel too bad today. I've been managing to get some of my supplement drinks down me without using the tube."

* * *

Many companies make specialised health supplements and drinks; during his recovery Michael used products from Fresenius Kabi, Enteral Nutrition, and Nutricia Advanced Medical Nutrition. In the US, the National Cancer Institute website has information about the importance of nutrition in cancer care. Your own health providers should be able to advise about nutrition for your condition.

* * *

"How can we help you, Mr Freeman?" a very attractive Nurse who he had not seen before stood at the door way of the waiting room where he had been waiting for twenty minutes. He explained his dilemma and the nurse smiled and stated that he would be seen shortly. Meanwhile he was offered a hot drink, which he surprisingly drunk without too much effort.

"We'll soon fix you up," said the nurse who had first spoken to him. "I'll just sort out all the equipment. "What's your date of birth?" He could not help thinking that if he had had a pound for every time he had been asked this question he would be a very rich man. But, as one Nurse explained to him a few weeks ago, mistakes can happen.

"That's hurting me," he cried as he felt the tube trying to find its way up his nose. "Can you please stop? It's very painful."

"Of course, we can try the other nostril if you prefer?" the young nurse smiled at him as she took out the tube and began to enter his left nostril.

"Sorry, that's just as bad." His eyes were watering and he couldn't recall a time when this procedure was so difficult.

"I'll go fetch the doctor and have a word. Won't be long," said the nurse, who quickly departed.

* * *

MOTORWAY – KEEP LEFT

"Look, doctor I've managed to swallow a cup of coffee earlier on. So I was thinking that as its Friday I'll try and manage without a tube. If I can't then I can always return to Bexley wing on Monday and see my regular staff." He was desperate not to have to repeat the previous scene.

"I don't see a problem with that. You know where we are if you run into any other problems, Mr Freeman. Just let us know," the doctor said reassuringly before she disappeared down the corridor.

"I'm off that flaming tube for a few days, Carole. Where can we go? I'm dying for a pint."

* * *

"This pint of real ale tastes like liquid gold, Carole."

"I guess you deserve it after all this time," remarked Carole. "Cheers, then."

"I've got another appointment with a Rehab team tomorrow". He slurped his first pint for over three months.

* * *

It didn't take long to find the Rehab Department based in Bexley Wing. He sat down in the waiting room after reporting to the receptionist. He only had to wait a few minutes before he was greeted by one of the Macmillan Nurses: "Hello, my name is Susan. Please can you complete this form so we can have an idea on where we all are?" Susan placed the form on his lap and left through the double doors.

He found himself in a room surrounded by three Nurses who all had pleasant and reassuring smiles. "I'll quickly introduce you to everyone, Michael," the nurse said. "Our role is to support you for the next few months. In a few minutes we'll have to weigh you. We don't want you to lose too much weight."

"Do you know the time and date of my scan? I've not heard from anyone yet," he asked apprehensively.

"Don't worry; someone will get in touch with you soon".

"I'm grateful for all your help," he said as he left the room feeling better than he had for a long time. One of the team was a dietician who gave him some valuable advice on what he could eat.

The phone call came a week later. The man on the other end of the phone explained in a reassuring tone that he would have to stop eating six hours before the scan. He was given other instructions, and assured that a letter would soon follow the phone call.

(The PET/CT scan or Positron Emission Tomography-Computed Tomography scan of the body; this procedure was completed by 'Alliance Medical' a private company outsourced by the NHS.)

"Carole, that was awful," he remarked as he gulped down half a bottle of water.

"Why, what's happened," Carole asked.

"I was placed in this room first, so I could be injected with what was described as a 'mildly radioactive tracer'. Not very pleasant, but I've had it before, if you remember?" She nods. "Then they took my chewing gum and water off me and I had to lie inside a long tunnel. My mouth started to feel like a cardboard box. I had to concentrate really hard to keep still, and I nearly stopped the procedure from finishing. But I kept telling myself that it was important to try and let it finish, we need to know if all the treatment has worked. One of the nurses told me that someone would give me a drink of water, but I guess they couldn't just stop. I must have been lying there gasping for thirty minutes."

"Well we'll hopefully get some results soon," remarked Carole. "I'm dying to go to the loo. It's also difficult waiting while you are looking after the coats and valuables."

"I'm ready for a pint and something to eat. Let's get off to the pub. I'm hungry." He gratefully took his coat from Carole who had been sent into the treatment area to collect him. "I'm glad that's over."

*   *   *

"I've found another person who does acupuncture," explained Carole. "She is a friend of Angela's, so she should be OK."

"I'll give her a ring. It will be good to try someone who lives nearer. Must try something to sort my mouth out it's driving me mad, especially at night."

*   *   *

"That was interesting, Carole. Linda, the acupuncturist has recommended a Chinese Herbalist. Apparently she has a relative who has used him and had some positive results from the treatment."

"Might be worth a try," said Carole.

"I might drive down that way tomorrow," he said, wondering if this option would help.

Acupuncture: known to be a remarkably safe treatment for all kinds of common problems - has been used in cancer to help relieve common symptoms such as pain, sleep and relaxation problems, or the nausea and sickness accompanying chemotherapy. Used in China for 2000 years, it has adapted into western medicine on a scientific basis as an effective addition to conventional treatments.
See "British Acupuncture Council"
www.acupunture.org.uk

"Look at these herbs the Chinese Herbalist has given me, Carole. Not cheap." He thrust a white paper bag full of different kinds of plants and herbs onto the kitchen side board. "I've got to boil the contents of the bag and drink the juice twice a day after meals. It's

51

interesting to watch him mixing of all the various ingredients together and then place them all into seven separate bags. I've to go back next week. He promised I'll feel some results in a couple of weeks."

"Worth a try, I guess... but they don't half smell," replied Carole. "I'm really not sure your stomach will cope with all that right now."

A few hours later, he had to admit she was right.

*   *   *

Carole asked: "What were the results of the PET scan?"

"I've to go back and have another scan in three months' time."

"Why, what's the problem?"

"The scan showed that there were still some little bits and pieces hanging around. The doctor felt the treatment needed more time to do its job."

"Very frustrating, I guess?"

"It is what it is. But I'm not looking forward to having another of those scans."

"What happened last time?"

"It's my dry mouth. I'm not allowed water or chewing gum, so it was very uncomfortable."

"Well, best to keep thinking positive, I guess."

"Easier said..."

"Let's hope it's not their way of telling me that something is seriously wrong!" remarked Carole.

*   *   *

Several months later, Michael and Carole had a consultation with the oncologist to discuss the results of various tests recommended as a result of the latest scan. The oncologist noticed a few vague shadows and blobs dotted around Michael's body, but the large blob that was in Michaels neck had disappeared. Michael's bowel area also received a full MOT, although a small dot was seen in the vicinity of his liver.

"I can offer you a biopsy if you like," the oncologist explains, "But it could be a bit messy as you are on warfarin and there might be lots of blood. There's no guarantee that they will get a sample either, as the blob is so small."

Michael's reply was well rehearsed: "I'm going to Portugal for two weeks. I would like to make a follow up appointment sometime in November when we get back. I don't want any more tests at the moment."

The oncologist replied: "I'm treating you, not the images on a screen and you look very well to me. Enjoy your life, Michael."

"Don't worry. We will!"

*   *   *

A SUMMARY OF THE STORY SO FAR

Michael was diagnosed with Prostate cancer in 2006. He found it difficult to realise that he was not a star in a Soap Opera and that the situation was "real life". He was referred to a Counsellor at "The Robert Ogden Centre" who helped him come to terms with the diagnosis; he continues to receive help from the Centre.

In November 2012 Michael arranged an appointment with his local GP after noticing a lump on the left side of his face. The doctor on duty diagnosed Mumps. This lump wanted to stay around, so Michael returned to his regular GP who referred him to the Assessment Centre at the hospital. He was sent home with a course of antibiotics and told to stay indoors as he might be infectious.

The doctor on duty also advised him to see his local dentist who was so concerned she quickly referred him to the Leeds Dental Hospital. The team based at the Dental Hospital took three painful biopsies; none of these revealed a diagnosis. Therefore, no treatment plan could be advised. The specialist noticed that Michael had serious heart problems, so a small operation to discover the nature of the tumour was not recommended. Michael was relieved that he wouldn't have to be admitted to hospital. He consequently went into denial.

The specialist is also part of a team that includes other doctors, plus a team of nurses. They arranged for an MRI Scan which revealed a large tumour situated just below Michael's tongue. Michael and his partner attended a meeting of all the medical professionals involved in his case in March, 2013, where it was concluded that no treatment could be offered as no clear sample of the tumour had been obtained. Michael was extremely happy about the prospect of going home and getting on with his life.

However, he was referred to a nurse based at the local hospice, who provided him and his Partner with on-going support. A bed was reserved whilst the couple began to make the necessary arrangements.

Michael decided to forget that anything was wrong as he was not in any pain and he had a full diary of events which included a holiday in Croatia. Towards the end of this holiday in July 2013 Michael began to notice that his throat felt sore and he developed a chesty cough. Michael returned to the team oncologist who convinced Michael that he should do something and quickly. Michael agreed to a second "true cut Biopsy" (long needle) after a second scan revealed that a small amount of the tumour had moved towards his left lymph gland.

A treatment plan could now begin…

Note: If, like Michael, you like to treat yourself with a holiday at times like this, and you want something a little special, you might like to consider Nomadic Thoughts (Worldwide Travel) www.nomadicthoughts.com

I survived this period by writing some poems
and trying to be hopeful about the
outcome.
I also enlisted all my contacts who
promised to place Michael inside a healing
circle.
One day, I began to watch a spider that
had started to build a web on the handle
on our car door. He (or maybe, she) had
plenty of hope...

SPIDERS
Casting lines
Web structures creating form
Weaving a strength
A way of coping

Gossamer threads
Connect to granite walls
Holding steady now
Casting patterns of infinite beauty

Safety within;
The intertwining of miracles;
Spinning
Through the fear
Holding us,
Catching hope...

*   *   *

RETURN TO THE AIRPORT

"Will all passengers on flight 565 please report to the reception desk at Terminal One." The echo of this announcement boomed across the airport. He picked up his bags and reluctantly left the Reality Lounge.

"What's going on?" he thought." I bet it's a waste of time, but I'd better go."

He stood staring blankly at the large window at the side of the terminal. He grimaced as he witnessed a plane take off to its unknown destination.

"Your flight won't be too long," he was politely informed by the receptionist at the flight desk. "The spare part has now arrived, so it shouldn't be too long. Tomorrow's Airlines apologise for any delay."

"I'll wait a bit longer, I guess." He rechecked his ticket, passport and boarding pass. Suddenly feeling the chill, he thrust his hand in his pockets. He slumped back onto his seat, feeling that he could be in for a long wait.

*   *   *

POSTSCRIPT

December 2014

At his last appointment with his oncologist Michael was informed that the tumour in his neck had disappeared. It seems that the treatment plan was successful; Michael is left with a few long term side effects but is determined to live life fully. He is in the process of booking more holidays...

ABOUT THE AUTHOR

Michael served twelve years in the Royal Navy, including five years on submarines. After this he spent his working life (1972 -2008) supporting children and adults who had been referred to Social Services and Voluntary Agencies. Initially a residential carer, he has also fostered eleven children with severe learning disabilities and is currently a 'shared life carer' for an adult who has lived with his family for twenty years.

Michael met his second partner Carole in 1989; they subsequently married in 1991, making a home for their respective children from their previous marriages. They both managed to study for their respective degrees while fostering; Michael obtained a 2.1 in Play work which broadened his thinking and career in all sorts of ways. He began to write poetry and books for children eight years ago.

He and Carole described their experience of fostering disabled children in '***Angels Are Not Just for Christmas***' published by Barney Books, £6.99. Michael is presently working on part one of a humorous autobiography '***Don't Lose Your Paddle***' describing his time spent on submarines and surface ships. He also created a series of children's stories, featuring an eleven year old girl who is a wheelchair user, for teachers who wish to introduce an inclusive agenda to children aged 4-10. The stories are available on an audio CD, '***Legends of Cyber Land***', £9.99

**Publications above available from
michaelfreeman175@gmail.com**